THE DEVELOPMENT
OF THE INFANT

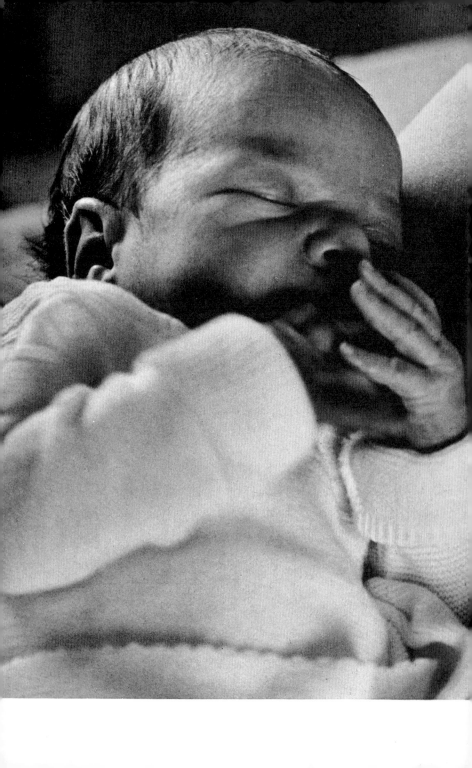

THE DEVELOPMENT
OF THE INFANT

the first year of life in photographs

Mark van Blankenstein
Ursula R. Welbergen
J.H. de Haas

WILLIAM HEINEMANN MEDICAL BOOKS LTD
LONDON

This study was compiled at the Department
of Social Hygiene of the Netherlands Institute
for Preventive Medicine, Leiden, under the
supervision of Prof. Dr. J. H. de Haas

First Published in the UK 1975
Reprinted 1978
© William Heinemann Medical Books Ltd 1975 UK Edition

ISBN 0 433 03235 9

Photoset, printed and bound
in Great Britain by
REDWOOD BURN LIMITED
Trowbridge & Esher

Contents

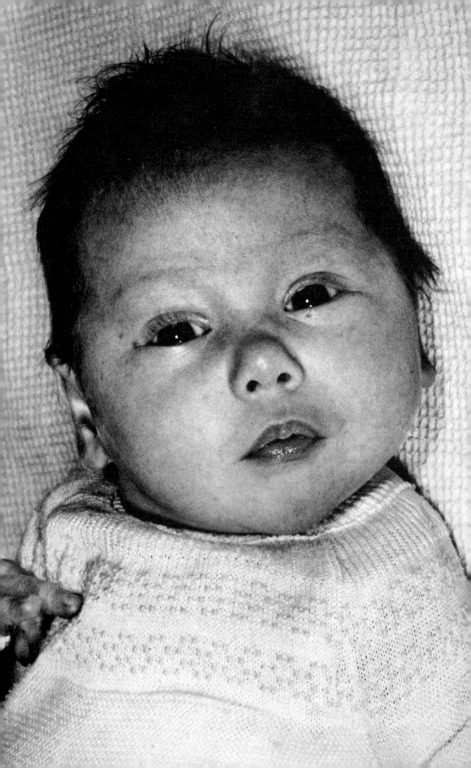

Foreword

This series of photographs of infant development was chosen from a collection built up by two students working at the Department of Health of the Netherlands Institute for Preventive Medicine, Leiden: Ursula Welbergen and Mark van Blankenstein. Together they have gathered a wealth of material and given form to the explanatory diagrams, which have been added to the photographs.

Mark van Blankenstein was the spiritual father of the photographs. The directions of Ursula Welbergen had the object of indicating which achievements of the infant were suitable for the photographic record of development.

The observations were compared with (medical) publications on infant development which have appeared in other countries.

The concept of this work is based on my experience during many years in the study of child development in different parts of the world.

Thanks to the co-operation and interest of mothers and fathers it was possible to build up a regular sequence of photographs at short intervals of the youngest member of the family in his habitual environment. The writers are grateful to the parents.

This atlas of infant development is dedicated to the dramatis personae, unconscious as they may be of the part they have played.

Leiden, 1972   J. H. de Haas

Two week old infant

Preface

This little book was published many years ago in both Dutch and French. The teachers of our courses abroad and we ourselves have used it for many years to teach normal child development. We have always regretted that no English translation existed.

Its advantages are that it is a real picture book, beautifully photographed and intelligently arranged, in trimesters, and explaining what happens at the beginning and towards the end of each one. Furthermore, it follows child development not only in a longitudinal direction but all bears a closer relationship to the well-known overlap of various aspects of this development by juxtaposing the various motor abilities appearing at the same time. This is an absolute precondition for an understanding of the various types of deviation found in abnormal conditions such as cerebral palsy, autism and mental retardation.

It should prove of great value to all those interested in normal and deviant child development.

Karel and Berta Bobath

Introduction

In the first year of life a human being evolves from a more or less helpless new born baby to a child that crawls or walks. Like every biological process this "miracle" occurs in all human beings in a comparable fashion. This aspect of infant development is illustrated by a series of photographs.

These pictures were taken with development in mind, which means that the medically trained photographer attempted to observe and record new functions at the earliest possible stage. The untrained observer will, however, tend to notice these new aptitudes at a later stage of their evolution.

Only a few children were followed up for these photographs and it is not proposed that they represent an average. With the aid of only these examples it is impossible to diagnose a retardation or advance in the development of any given child.

It is not intended to imply that an infant is able to lift his head at six weeks, sit up at 26 weeks, and walk at 52 weeks. On the contrary, the object is to demonstrate the continuity and regularity in development and to display the various functions both separately and in their mutual relation without rigid chronological schedules.

In this work the main emphasis is laid on motor development. It is impossible to isolate motor from mental development in infants. Mental reactions, however, are difficult to register photographically while objective interpretation from photographs is still more difficult.

Although the various components of development form a central theme, motor activities make the greatest impression on the observer and are also suitable for visual representation.

Added to the photographs are a number of explanatory diagrams.

Photographs, diagrams and text in close correlation, attempt to give an insight into the commonplace, but marvellous, happening known as biological development.

The evolution of eye movements and manipulation are represented separately.

Some understanding of growth and development in the first year stimulates the tendency towards observation, which is common to all parents.

A growth diagram is also printed, compiled from recent data on weight and height of many children in the first year of life. In this diagram a number of the most important functions have been indicated.

Insight into the process of development stimulates better infant-care. This should be given in a form adapted to the biological development of the individual infant and not in a rigid manner.

This work, in which photographs speak more than the brief text, has as its objects:

—to acquaint parents with the development of the young child

—to base infant-care more firmly on biological insight than was the case up till now

—to stimulate interest for growth and development of the child.

The publication of this series of photographs of infant development aims above all at the greater happiness of parents and their children.

These four pictures each represent an important phase in development during the first year.

During the first quarter the child starts to lift up its head.

During the second quarter sitting with help is gradually achieved.

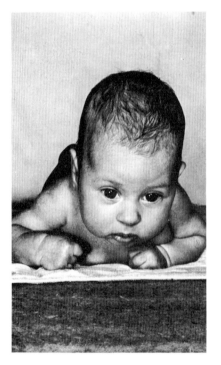

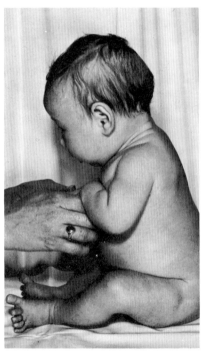

During the third quarter the child can pull to standing but with variable success.

During the fourth quarter the child starts to crawl, tries to walk in its playpen. It is able to take a few steps with help.

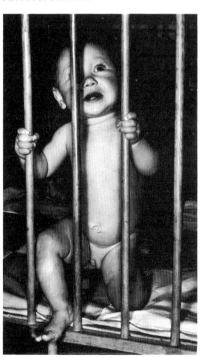

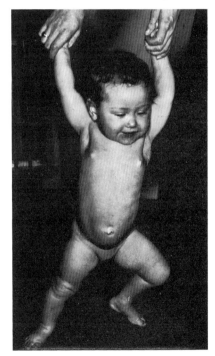

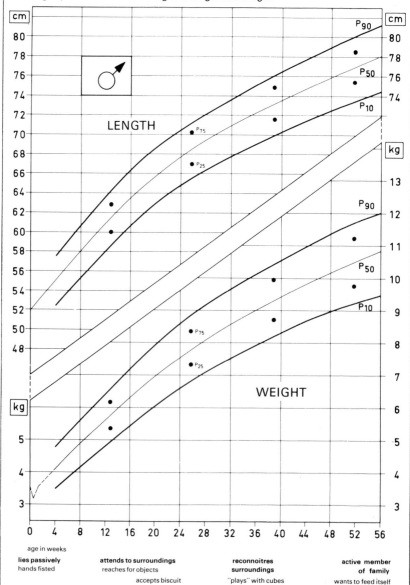

GROWTH CURVES

boys

length and weight of 80% of the boys fall within the heavy drawn lines;
the lightly drawn lines are averages of length and weight

LENGTH

WEIGHT

age in weeks

lies passively	attends to surroundings	reconnoitres	active member
hands fisted	reaches for objects	surroundings	of family
	accepts biscuit	"plays" with cubes	wants to feed itself

14

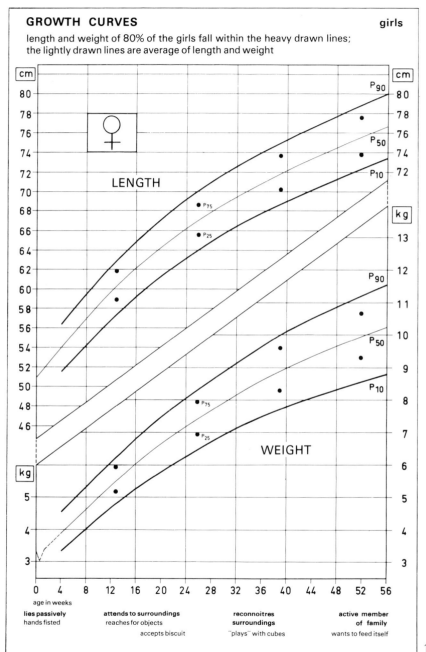

GROWTH CURVES

girls

length and weight of 80% of the girls fall within the heavy drawn lines;
the lightly drawn lines are average of length and weight

LENGTH

WEIGHT

age in weeks

lies passively	attends to surroundings	reconnoitres	active member
hands fisted	reaches for objects	surroundings	of family
	accepts biscuit	"plays" with cubes	wants to feed itself

15

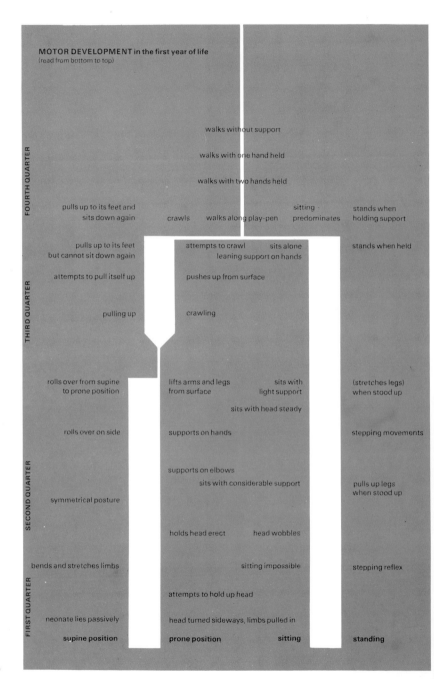

MOTOR DEVELOPMENT in the first year of life
(read from bottom to top)

FOURTH QUARTER

walks without support

walks with one hand held

walks with two hands held

pulls up to its feet and sits down again · crawls · walks along play-pen · sitting predominates · stands when holding support

THIRD QUARTER

pulls up to its feet but cannot sit down again · attempts to crawl · sits alone leaning support on hands · stands when held

attempts to pull itself up · pushes up from surface

pulling up · crawling

SECOND QUARTER

rolls over from supine to prone position · lifts arms and legs from surface · sits with light support · (stretches legs) when stood up

sits with head steady

rolls over on side · supports on hands · stepping movements

supports on elbows

sits with considerable support · pulls up legs when stood up

symmetrical posture

holds head erect · head wobbles

FIRST QUARTER

bends and stretches limbs · sitting impossible · stepping reflex

attempts to hold up head

neonate lies passively · head turned sideways, limbs pulled in

supine position · **prone position** · **sitting** · **standing**

Motor Development

The photographs have been grouped according to the diagram (shown on the opposite page) illustrating the most significant achievements from birth until the first birthday.

In this diagram the first year is divided into four quarters, not because these are separate periods, but because events occur so swiftly in the first year of development that it cannot be considered as one period.

It is a mistake to adhere strictly to an age table when judging development; each child has his own rate of development. This, however, does not invalidate the fact that the child arrives at the different stages according to a regular sequence. The infant can lift his head before he can push himself up on his hands and can stand before he can walk.

In this diagram the prone and supine positions and sitting and standing have been distinguished as the most important elements of motor development.

The supine and prone positions are the only possible unaided postures for the young infant.

Sitting and standing—as demonstrated in various photographs—are only possible when the child is placed in these attitudes and supported.

Before the end of the first quarter, usually around the end of the second month, the infant is able to lift up his head from the prone position.

The child as yet has little contact with his surroundings.

The diagram demonstrates the continuity and regularity in development and is not a chronological table. Forwardness or retardation in development cannot be concluded from it.

In the second quarter the passive posture gradually changes into active movement and the infant begins to take notice of the world around him. When he hears his mother approaching or hears her talk he will wave his arms and legs about and smile.

At the end of the first half year the infant rolls from the supine into the prone position and pushes himself up on his hands. When stood up the child stretches his legs against the ground and bounces up and down. For sitting, light support is still essential.

At the beginning of the third quarter the supine position is no longer followed up in the diagram as the infant tends to attempt new activities—like pulling up and crawling—from the prone position. The supine position is only assumed when resting. Crawling and pulling up are now treated separately in the diagram as new functions.

Standing with support is achieved at the end of the third quarter. In these months sitting is a position in which many activities are carried out.

About the beginning of the fourth quarter the sequence of sitting—crawling—pulling up to his feet—walking along the play-pen and sitting down is completed. Nothing is safe when the child is about. He potters around the room and lays his hands on everything within reach.

During the fourth quarter the movements of locomotion become more co-ordinated. The child pulls himself up on his feet, stands and walks with support.

Shortly before or after his first birthday he takes his first independent steps. The infant has become a toddler.

Motor development

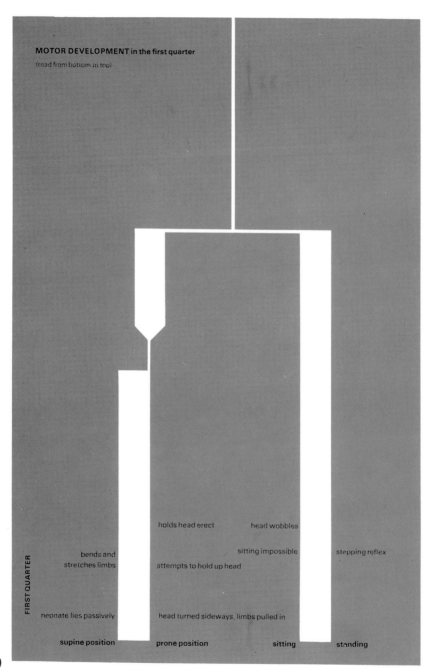

MOTOR DEVELOPMENT in the first quarter
(read from bottom to top)

FIRST QUARTER

holds head erect   head wobbles

bends and   sitting impossible   stepping reflex
stretches limbs   attempts to hold up head

neonate lies passively   head turned sideways, limbs pulled in

supine position   **prone position**   **sitting**   **standing**

First quarter

The characteristic attitude of the newborn is lying passively with arms and legs drawn up. This attitude is derived from the intra-uterine position.

After a few days the infant begins to bend and stretch his limbs.

During the first month of life, the movements in the knee and elbow joints increase.

When lying prone the child attempts to lift up his head, he succeeds for a short while with the head turned sideways.

Halfway through the first quarter the arm and leg movements become more powerful. The scope of movements in the shoulder and hip joints increases.

The baby lies with his feet touching the underlying surface, the arms next to the head. In the prone position the head is lifted up for a somewhat longer time than in the first few weeks.

At the end of the first quarter the infant kicks about so energetically that he rolls over on his side. Waving and kicking show a liveliness which can make it difficult to handle the child, in dressing for instance. The wholly passive existence is past.

Lying prone the head can be lifted for several minutes and held up in midline: It no longer turns sideways.

When sat up the baby assumes a slumped position, the head wobbling from side to side. When placed in standing position, the infant draws up his legs alternately as they touch the ground. This movement is a reflex, not to be confused with the "real" stepping movements which occur at the end of the first half year.

supine and prone position of the neonate

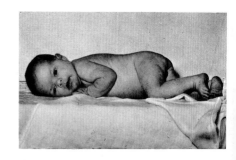

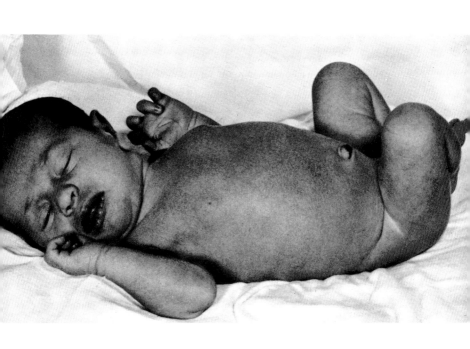

supine

bends and stretches limbs

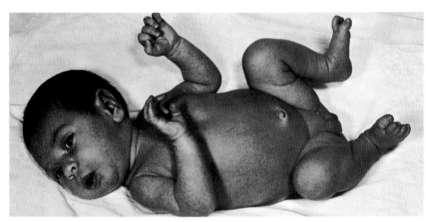

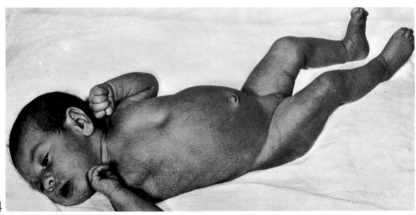

prone

raises head up for a few seconds

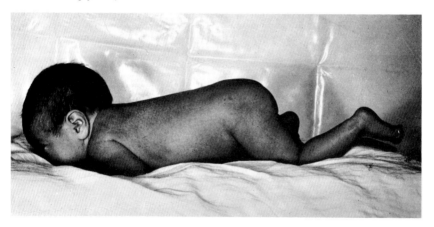

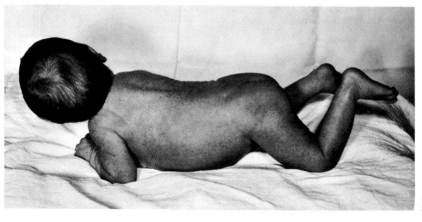

supine

above: asymmetrical posture
below: rolls over on side by kicking

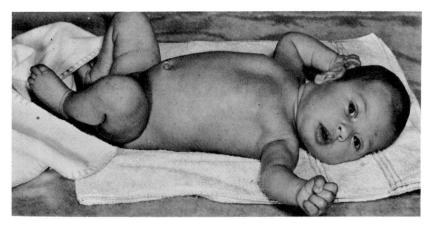

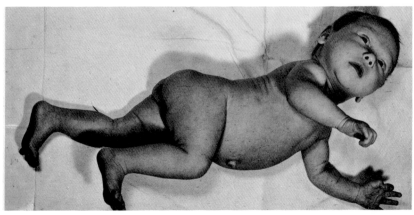

prone

above: raises head up for longer periods
below: raises head up straight in midline

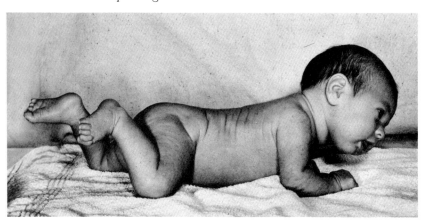

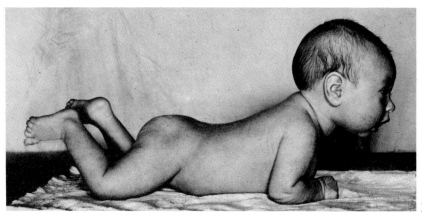

sitting

slumps when sat up

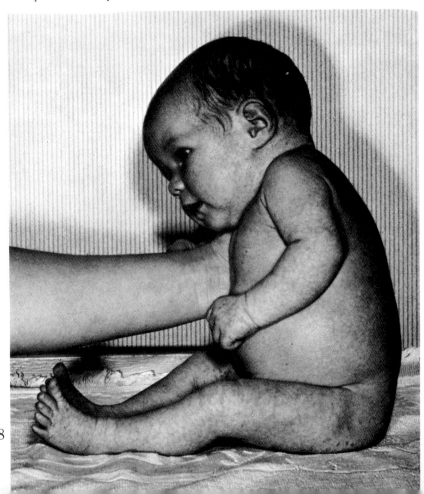

when pulled up the head lags less

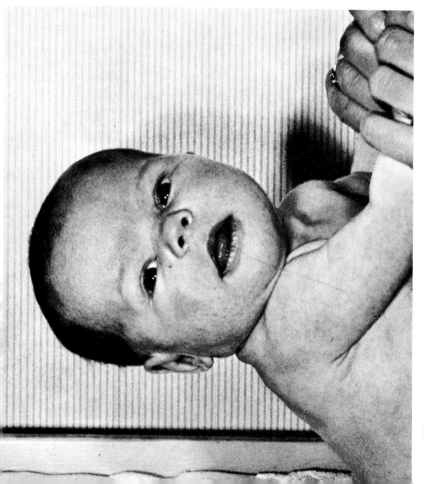

when stood up on a hard surface the result is . . .

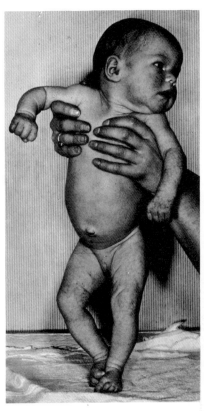

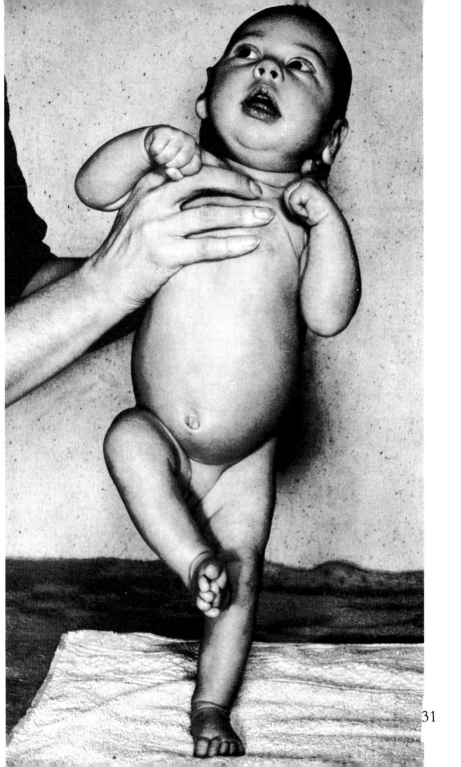

31

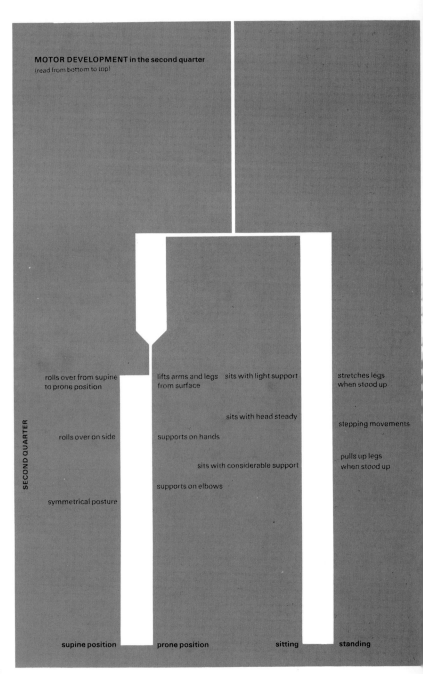

MOTOR DEVELOPMENT in the second quarter
(read from bottom to top)

SECOND QUARTER

rolls over from supine
to prone position

lifts arms and legs
from surface

sits with light support

stretches legs
when stood up

sits with head steady

stepping movements

rolls over on side

supports on hands

sits with considerable support

pulls up legs
when stood up

supports on elbows

symmetrical posture

supine position   **prone position**   **sitting**   **standing**

Second quarter

During the first half of the second quarter the child lies symmetrically in the supine position, looking straight up.

In the prone position he looks around with head raised, supporting himself on his elbows and later on his hands.

At the end of the second quarter activity increases considerably. The child notices his surroundings; lying on his back is no longer a satisfying posture. He tries to roll over and after a few weeks succeeds in doing this. The infant can now easily fall off the bed if not watched.

In the prone position great activity is displayed. The infant pushes himself up and can, supported by one hand, snatch at various objects. The limbs make swimming movements. The baby waves his arms and legs in the air, but cannot yet move about.

In the period between the first and second quarter the child, when sat up, cannot hold his head steady, but it wobbles less than previously. Sitting still requires considerable support. The baby has a tendency to fall forwards or sideways.

At the beginning of the second quarter the baby no longer draws up his legs alternately but both together when stood up.

At the end of the second quarter the infant can sit with slight support and hold his head erect.

When the child is pulled up by his hands he participates in the movement, and his head no longer lags behind. When stood up the child keeps his feet on the ground and bounces up and down or makes step-like movements.

Within the first half year the infant has evolved from a helpless new-born-baby into a person almost able to sit and to observe his surroundings.

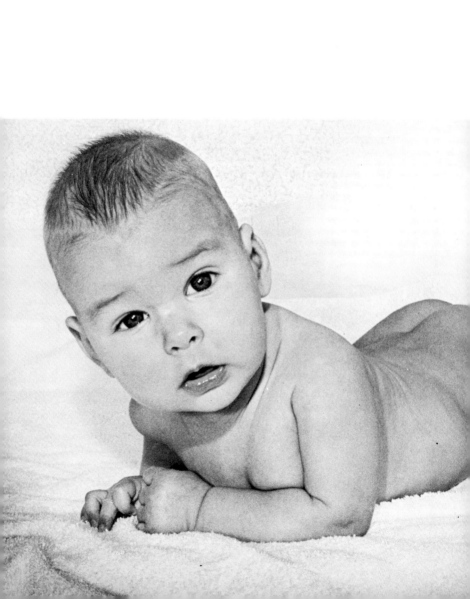

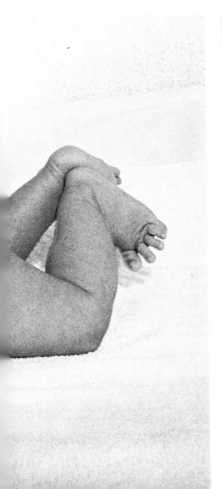

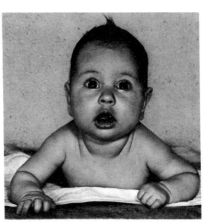

supine *symmetrical posture*
prone *head is held up, supports on fore-arms*

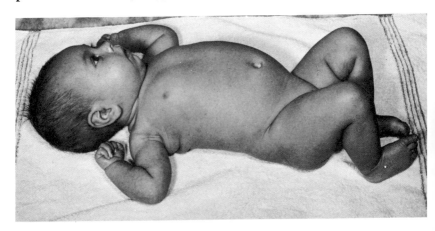

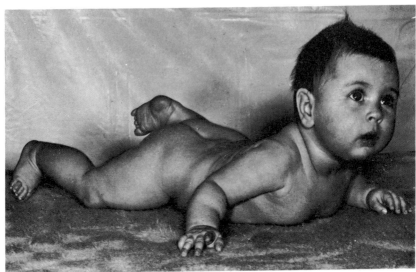

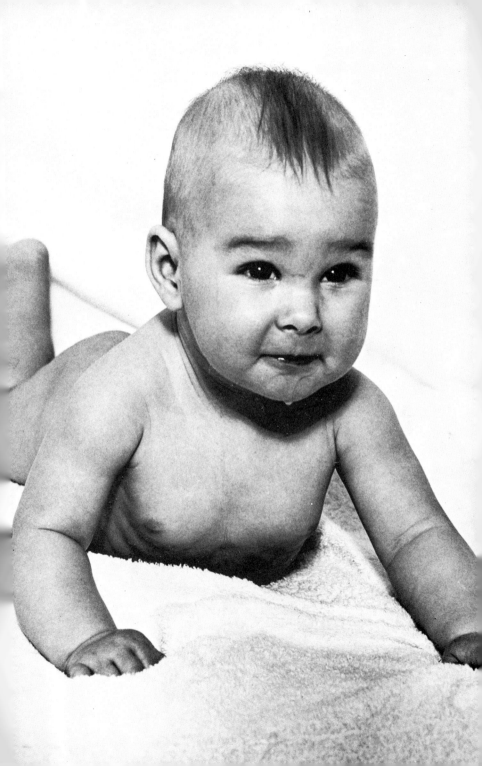

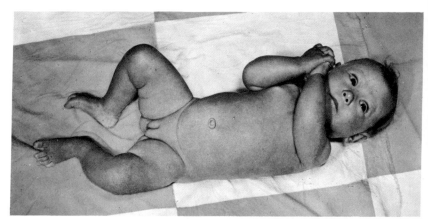

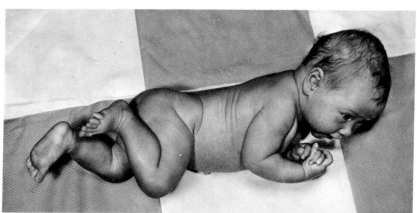

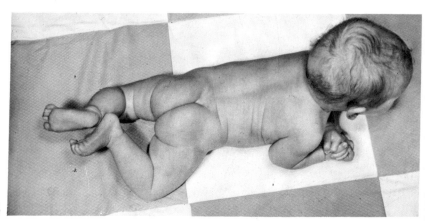

supine
*rolls over from
supine to prone position*

prone
rakes at objects

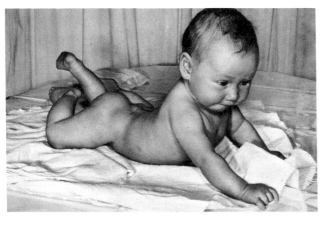

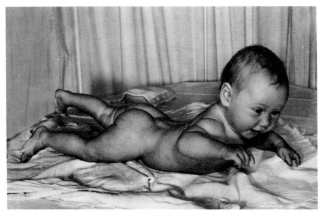

sitting

when pulled up the head is quite steady

sits with support

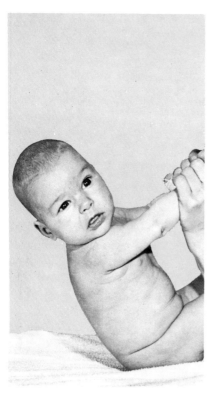
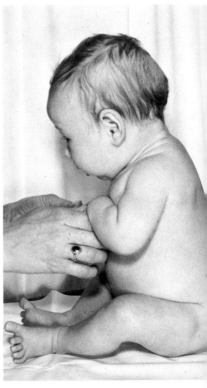

co-operates when sat up

sits with light support

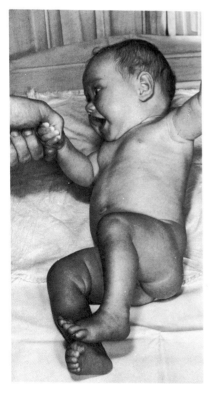
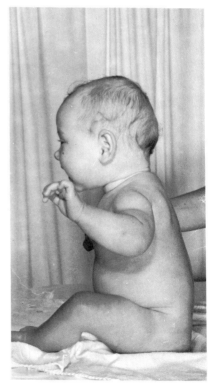

standing

pulls up legs when stood up on hard surface

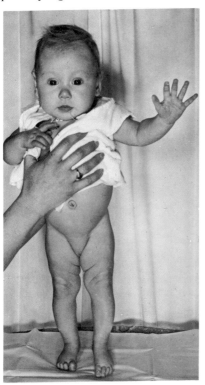 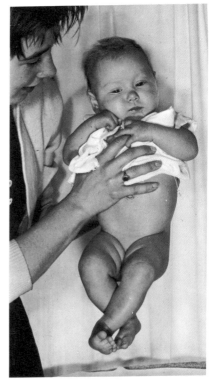

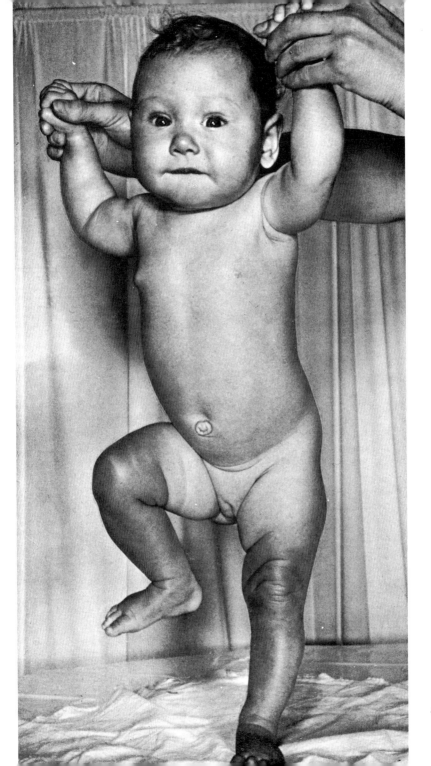

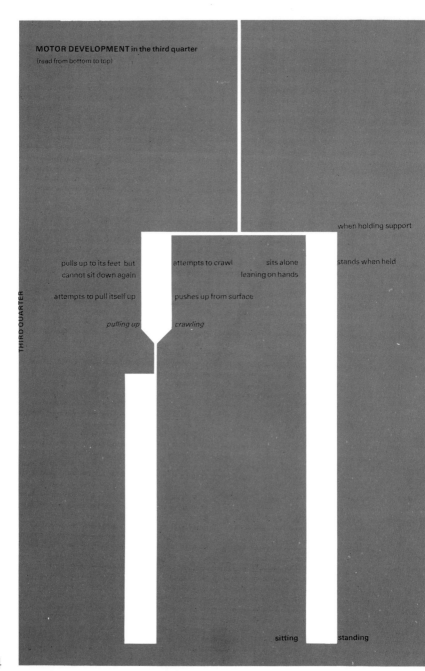

MOTOR DEVELOPMENT in the third quarter
(read from bottom to top)

THIRD QUARTER

when holding support

pulls up to its feet but   attempts to crawl   sits alone   stands when held
cannot sit down again   leaning on hands

attempts to pull itself up   pushes up from surface

pulling up   *crawling*

sitting   standing

44

Third quarter

The baby rolls over from the supine to the prone position and begins to explore his surroundings. From the latter position crawling and pulling up evolve. The supine position is no longer regarded as a separate function in the diagram.

As a first attempt at crawling the baby pushes his body up, drags himself along with his hands and lets himself fall on his chest. The eight to nine month-old baby mainly moves about by using his arms.

During the third quarter the child begins to pull himself up by the bars of the play-pen and hangs from them, but cannot stand.

When the child is seven or eight months old he can sit without being supported while leaning forward on his hands.

When standing, the child has to be supported by both hands.

At the transition from the third to the fourth quarter the infant sits, crawls, pulls himself up on his feet, stands and walks along the play-pen and sits down again. Most of these activities are initiated from the sitting position.

At this stage of motor development the functions originally differentiated are merged (in the diagram) as the child is able to integrate them.

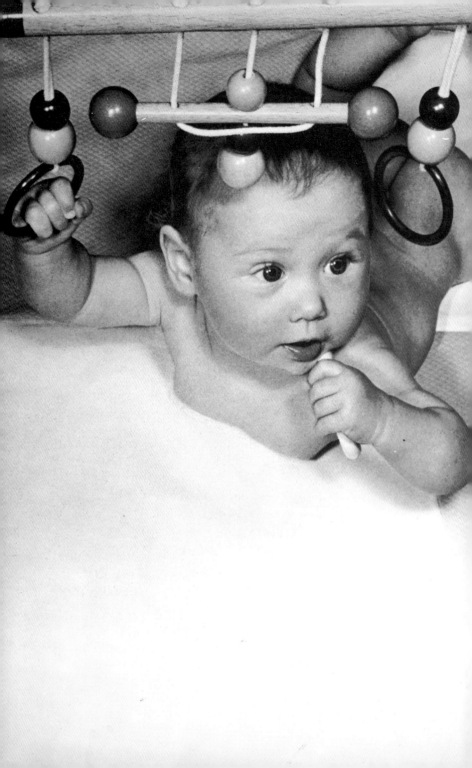

pulling up

crawling

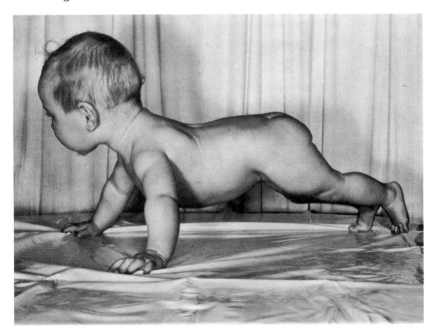

crawling

above: pushes up
below: supports on hands

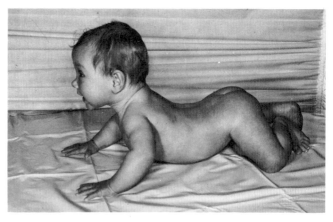

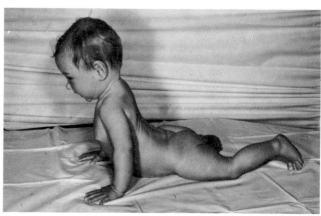

above: drags herself forwards
below: lets herself fall

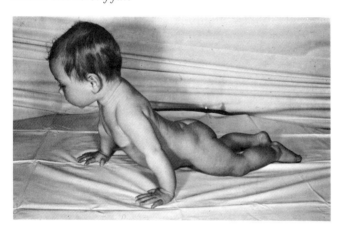

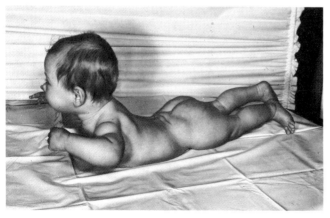

pulling up

pulls herself up to her feet

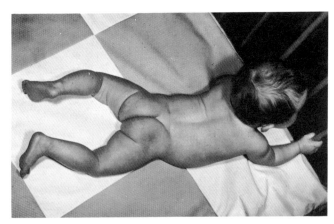

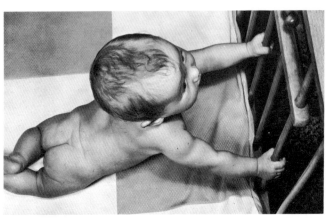

can't get down again

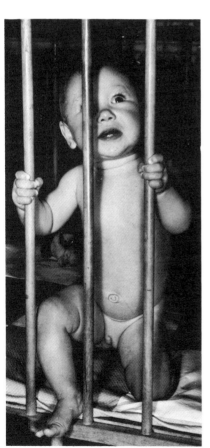 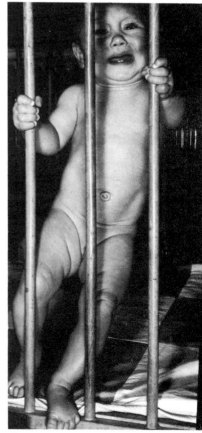

standing
stands with support
(bounces up and down)

sitting
sits alone, leaning on hands

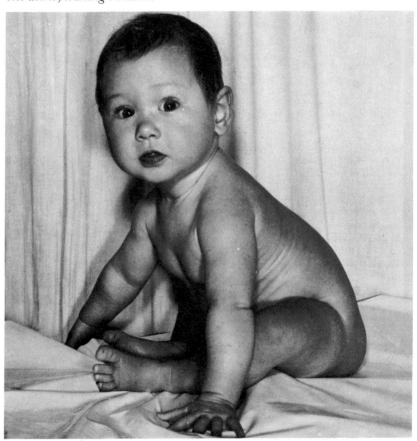

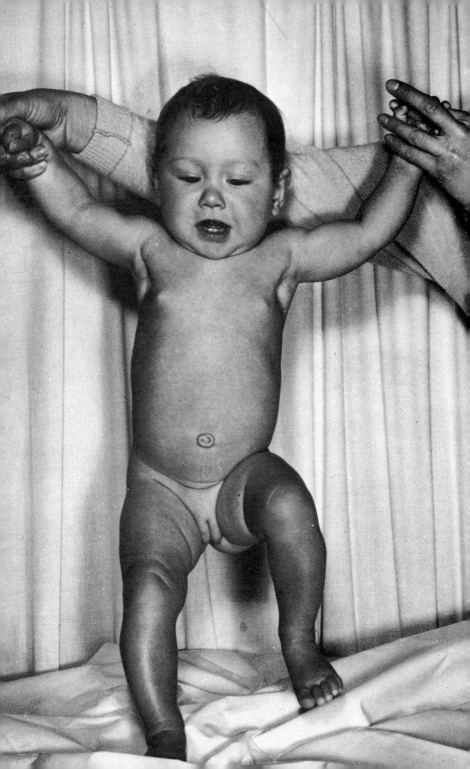

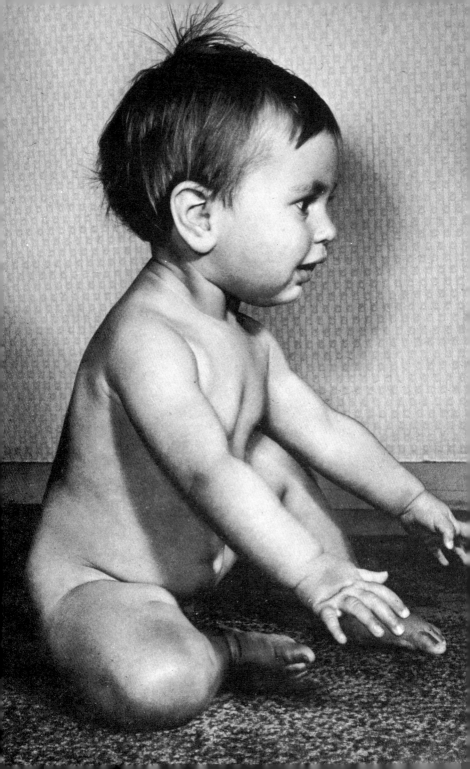

crawling
goes about on her seat

crawls on hands and knees

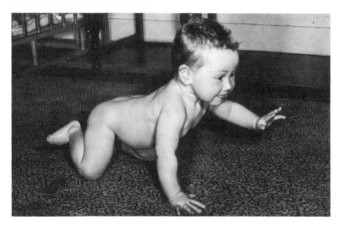

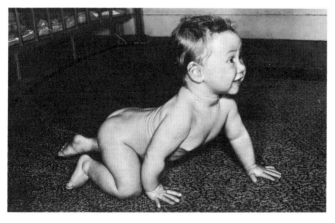

55

crawling

crawls on hands and feet

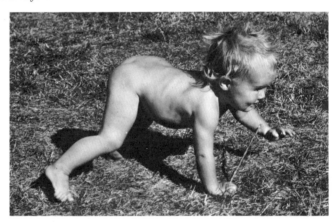

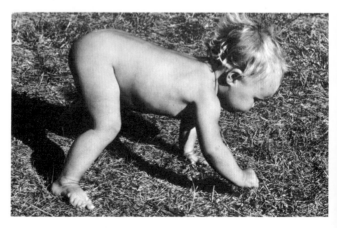

The cycle of standing—sitting—crawling—walking along the play-pen and standing pictured on the following pages, will often be completed when the child is between eight and ten months old.

The motor functions of one child in the second half of the third quarter may be as far developed as those of another child in the first half of the fourth quarter.

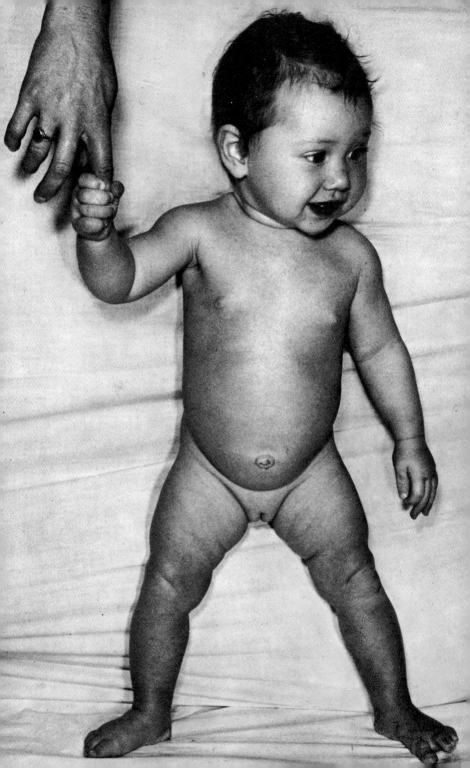

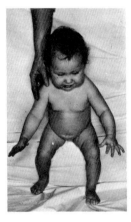

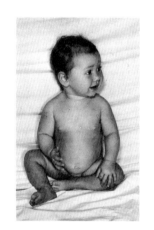

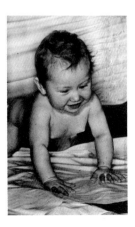

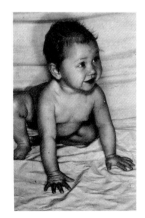

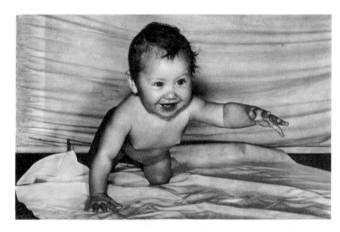

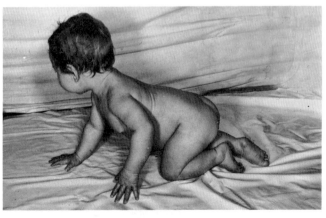

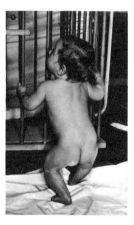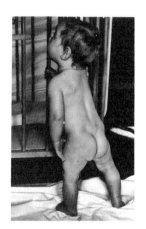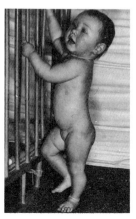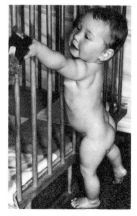

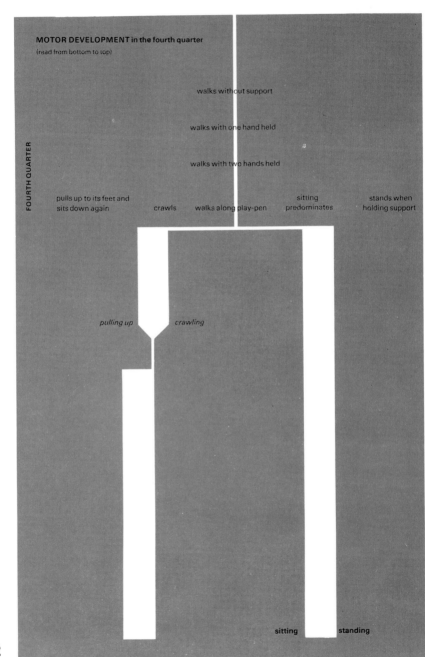

MOTOR DEVELOPMENT in the fourth quarter
(read from bottom to top)

FOURTH QUARTER

walks without support

walks with one hand held

walks with two hands held

pulls up to its feet and
sits down again

crawls   walks along play-pen

sitting
predominates

stands when
holding support

pulling up   *crawling*

sitting   **standing**

Fourth quarter

In the fourth quarter, locomotion becomes the most important motor function. At first the child moves about by crawling.

Many different methods of crawling are practised. Each child has his own style of crawling on hands and knees or on hands and feet. He also moves about on his buttocks.

In walking the child still needs to be held by both hands. Leaning forward he takes steps with legs wide apart. Gradually walking movements become more co-ordinated.

Round about his first birthday, the child walks supported by one hand. The first hesitant unsupported steps follow, in which the whole body is tense. After a few steps the child falters and sits down or stumbles.

A few months later (in the beginning of the second year of life) the young toddler walks with his body relaxed. His feet are gradually placed in a less straddled position.

walking

stands holding on with one hand

cannot walk with only one hand held

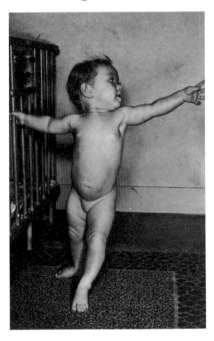

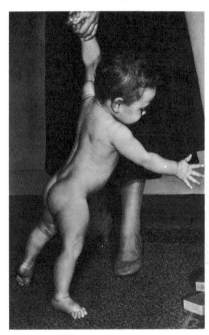

can walk with both hands held

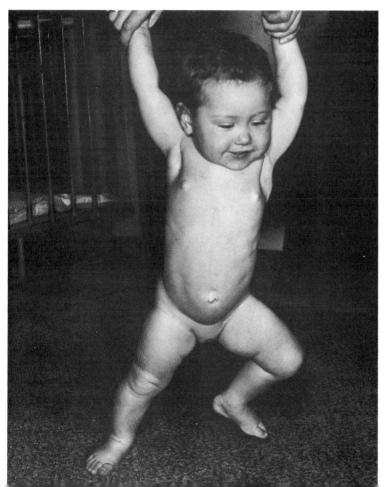

walking

walks with one hand held

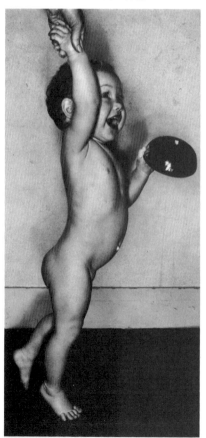

stands without support

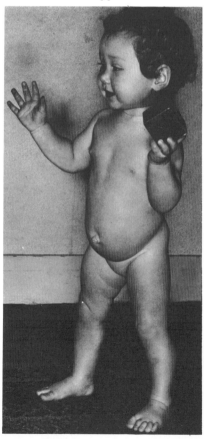

walks wide-legged

loses her balance

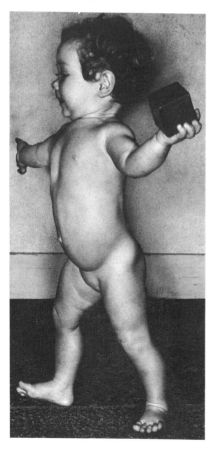

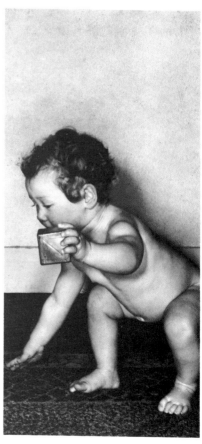

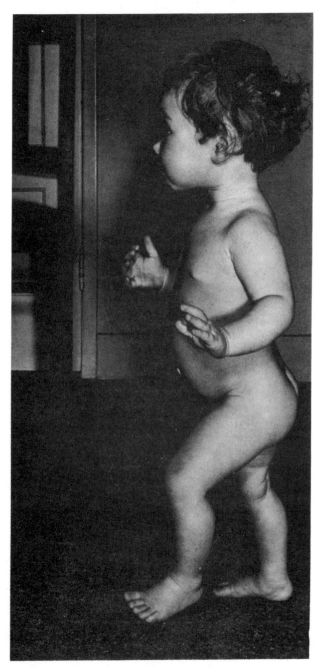

*walks
unsuppor
and relax*

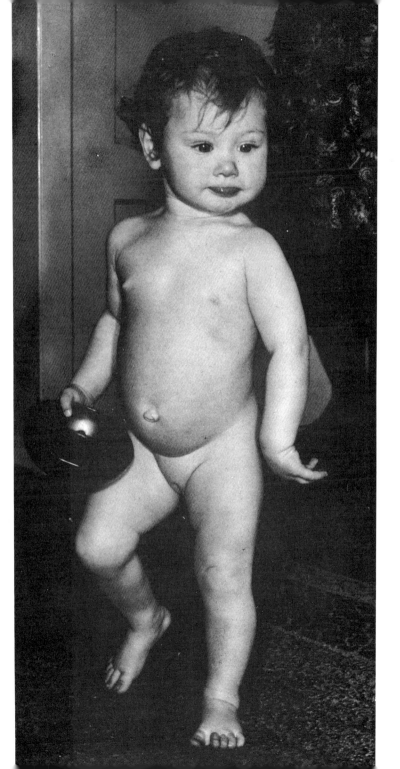

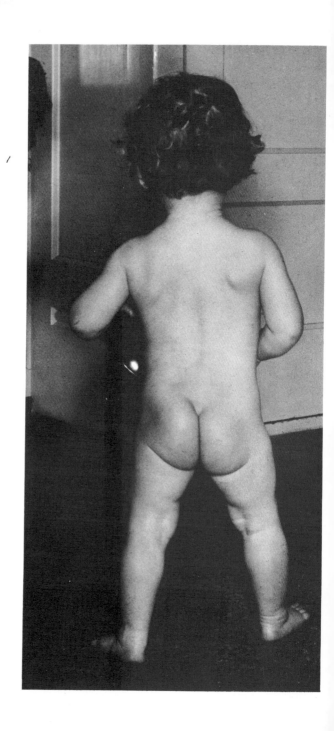

Development of eye and hand movements

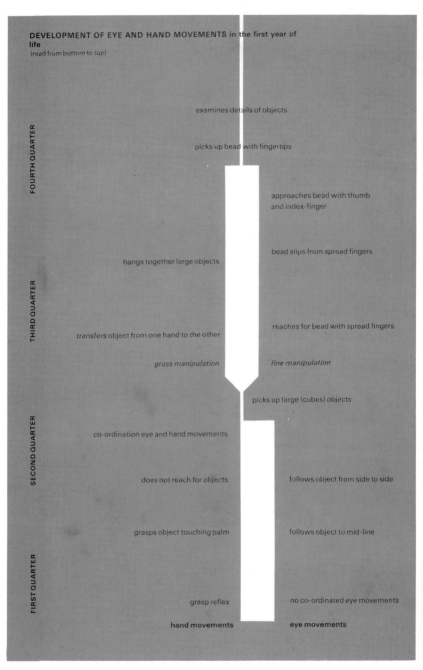

DEVELOPMENT OF EYE AND HAND MOVEMENTS in the first year of life
(read from bottom to top)

FOURTH QUARTER

examines details of objects

picks up bead with fingertips

approaches bead with thumb and index-finger

bead slips from spread fingers

THIRD QUARTER

bangs together large objects

transfers object from one hand to the other

reaches for bead with spread fingers

gross manipulation

fine manipulation

picks up large (cubes) objects

SECOND QUARTER

co-ordination eye and hand movements

does not reach for objects

follows object from side to side

grasps object touching palm

follows object to mid-line

FIRST QUARTER

grasp reflex

no co-ordinated eye movements

hand movements

eye movements

Development of eye and hand movements.

Eye and hand movements have been distinguished as separate functions in this diagram as the young infant cannot direct his hands to the objects he sees and therefore cannot grasp them.

Eye movements are not co-ordinated in the first few weeks. The infant cannot look at a particular object.
In the course of the second month the capacity for fixing objects with the eyes develops. The baby watches a moving object and follows it up to the vertical plane. As soon as it passes to the other side of this plane, however, it is lost from sight.
During the first quarter the hands are predominantly held fisted. Grasping is still reflex. When objects are placed in the palm of the hand they are grasped and held.

At the beginning of the second quarter the eyes follow a moving object from one side to the other. The infant can now turn his head from side to side.
During the second quarter the co-operation of eyes and hands emerges: the infant fixes objects with his eyes and stretches out his arms towards them, at first using two arms, and later only one. Large objects which can be contained by one hand are held, thumbed and sucked.

In the beginning of the third quarter, distinction is made in the diagram between the manipulation of small and large objects. Large objects are grasped and beaten together. The child attempts, in vain, to pick up beads

The diagram demonstrates the continuity and regularity in development and is not a chronological table. Forwardness or retardation in development cannot be concluded from it.

and marbles with scissor-like movements of the spread fingers.

In the fourth quarter the developing toddler starts to pick up small objects with the tips of his thumb and index-finger. When this function is developed the child examines the details of larger objects with his fingertips.

first quarter
fist clenched

second quarter
reaches for objects

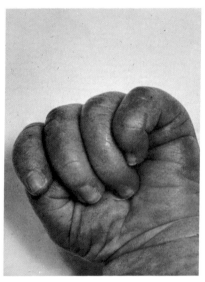
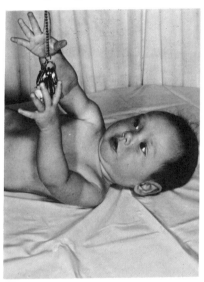

During the first and second quarters eye and hand movements develop independently, in the third and fourth quarter they are co-ordinated.

third quarter
handles large objects

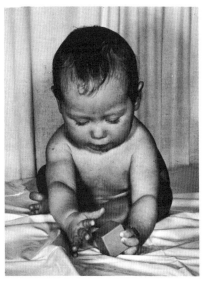

fourth quarter
fine manipulation

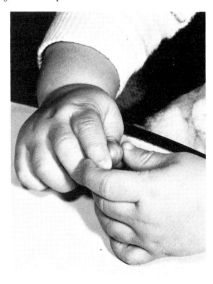

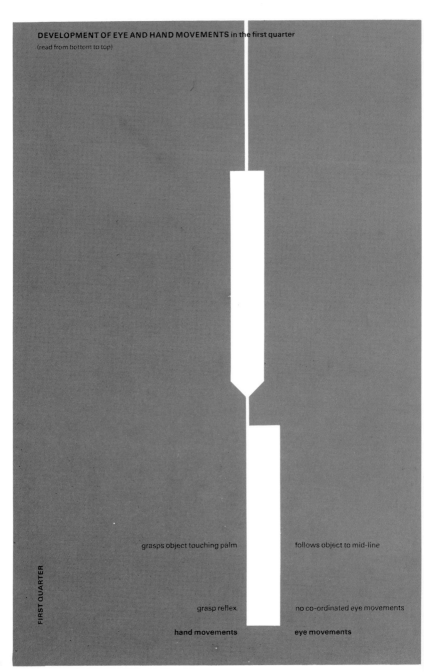

DEVELOPMENT OF EYE AND HAND MOVEMENTS in the first quarter
(read from bottom to top)

grasps object touching palm

follows object to mid-line

FIRST QUARTER

grasp reflex

no co-ordinated eye movements

hand movements

eye movements

76

First quarter
In the first weeks the hands are predominantly held clenched in a fist. When an object is placed in the palm of the hand it is grasped tightly and cannot be released voluntarily. Hand movements are involuntary, reflex actions. The eye movements are not yet co-ordinated, the baby cannot fix his gaze at a given spot.
The capacity for fixing the eyes on an object develops in the second month of life.

During the second to third month the baby is able to follow a moving object with both eyes. The head movements, however, are not sufficiently controlled to turn the head from one side to the other while following. He only follows the object until it is straight above his head; when it passes to the other side the infant loses it out of sight.
The baby can now fasten his eyes onto an object and follow it about, but does not yet reach for it with his hands.

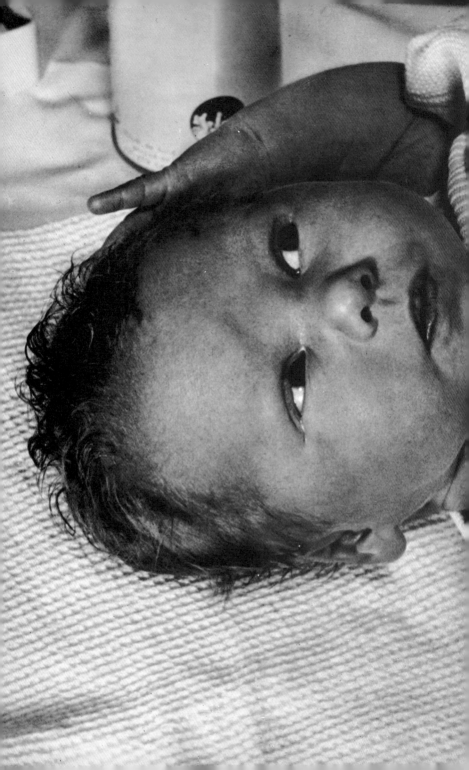

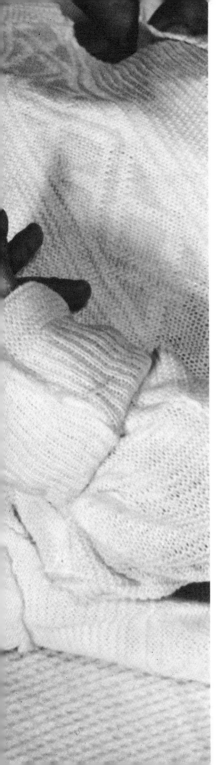
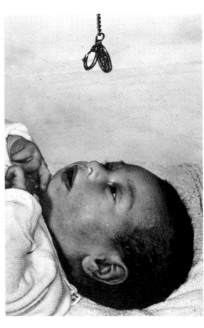

hand movements

fist clenched

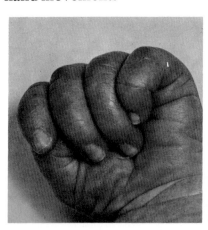

*hand grasps object
(grasping reflex)*

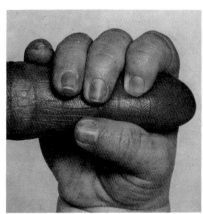

eye movements *undirected gaze*

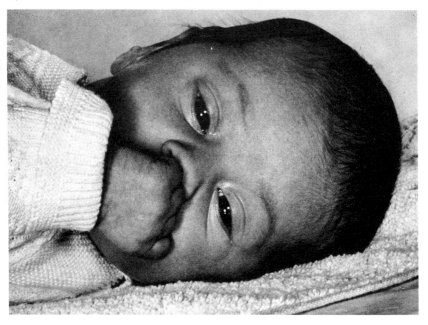

eye movements

follows object

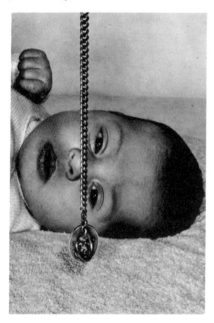

turns head . . .

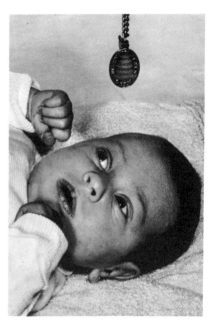

to mid-line

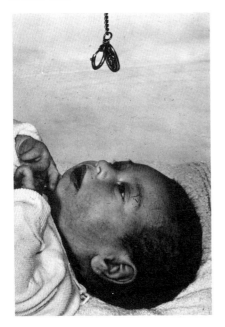

DEVELOPMENT OF EYE AND HAND MOVEMENTS in the second
quarter (read from bottom to top)

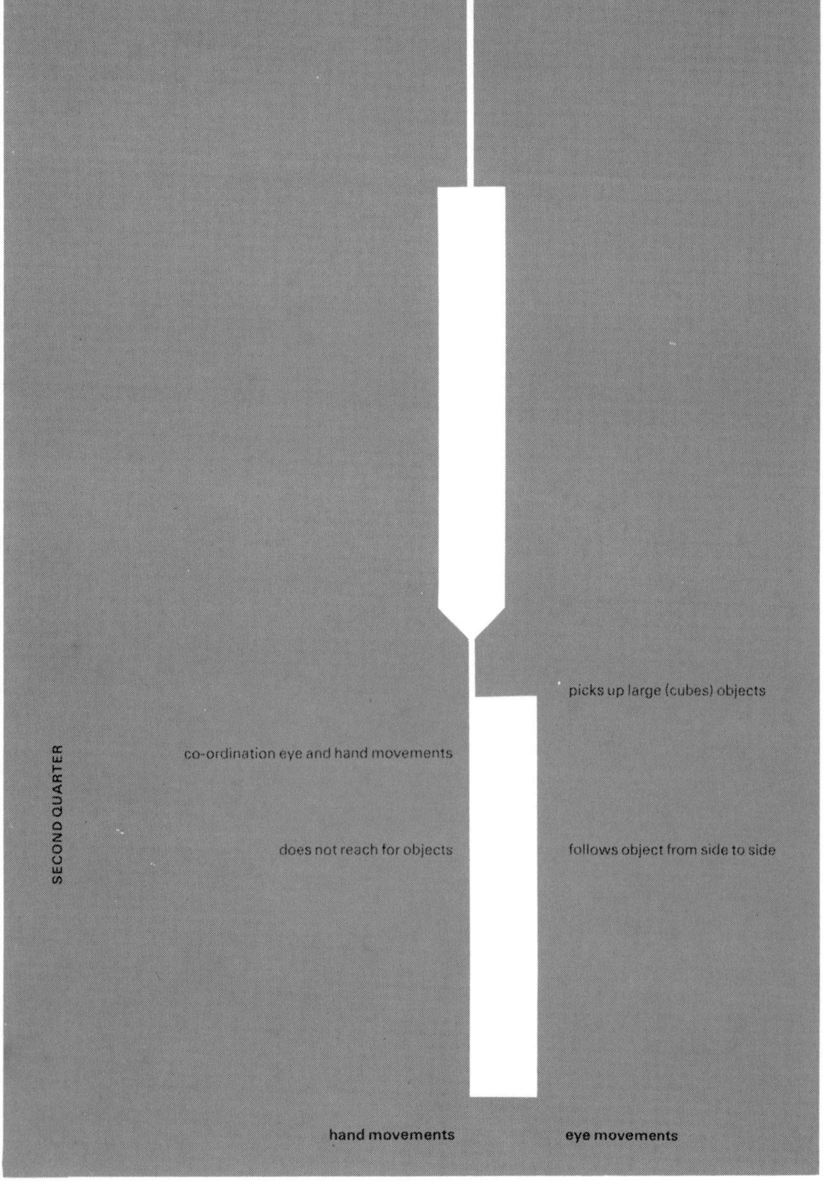

SECOND QUARTER

picks up large (cubes) objects

co-ordination eye and hand movements

does not reach for objects

follows object from side to side

hand movements

eye movements

Second quarter

At the beginning of the second quarter the infant is able to rotate his head sufficiently to follow an object from one side to the other. When an object is put into the baby's hand, it is clasped reflexly. Objects are mainly held by the last three fingers, thumb and index-finger hardly come into play.

In the course of the second quarter co-ordination between eye and hand movements is established. The infant stretches out his hands towards moving or stationary objects. At first both arms are used, later only one.
At the end of the second quarter the baby picks up objects. They should be small enough to be held in one hand. These 'toys' are inspected, handled and suddenly released.

The first half year sees the infant developing into an (almost) sitting child. The interplay between hands and eyes develops. This leads to the ability to reach for and to accept objects.

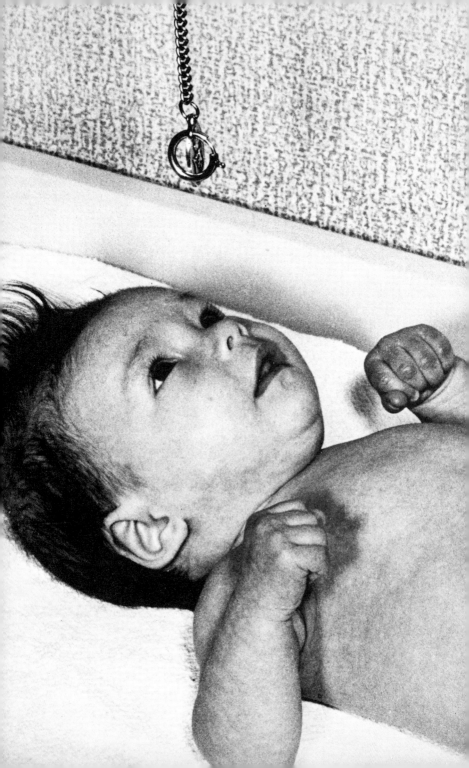

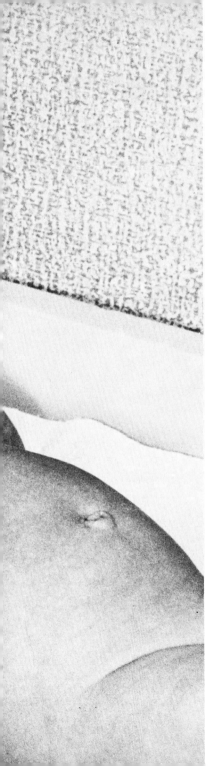

eye movements

when following objects

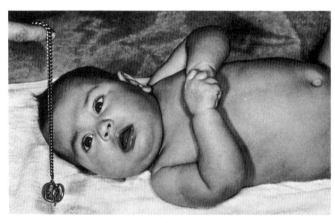

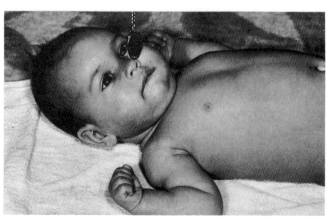

turns head from one side to the other

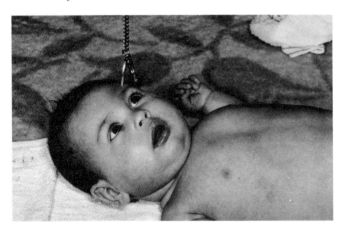

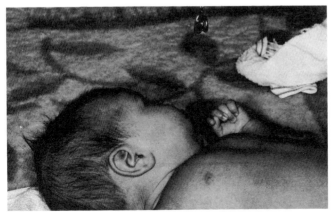

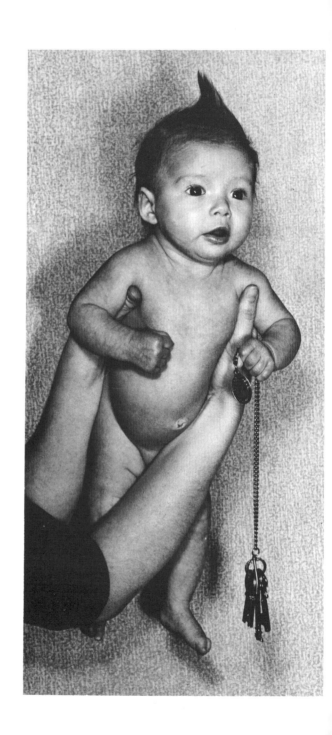

hand movements
grasp and holds an object put into palm

*grasps with last
three fingers*

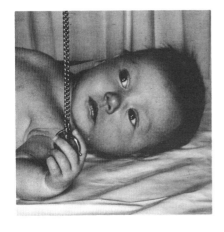 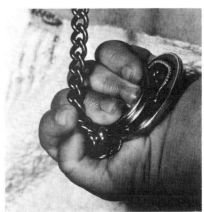

co-ordination of eye and hand movements

grasps object with one hand

reaches for object with both hands

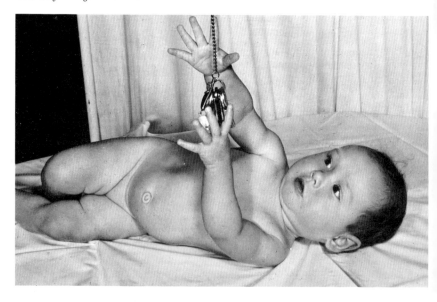

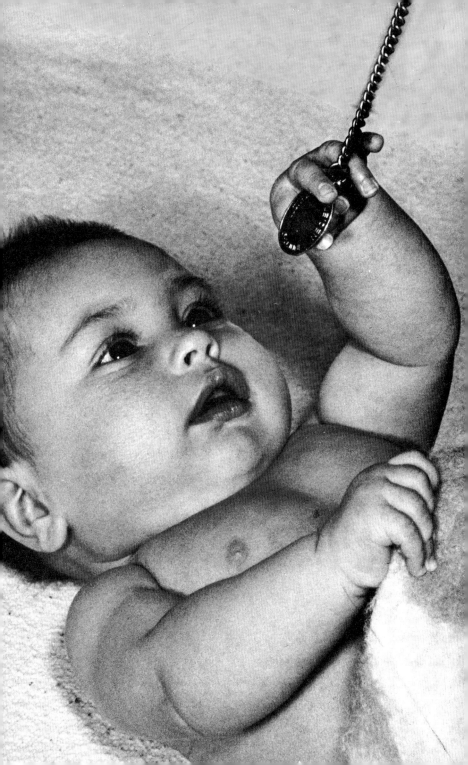

co-ordination of eye and hand movements

grasps and examines object

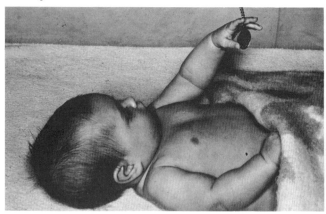

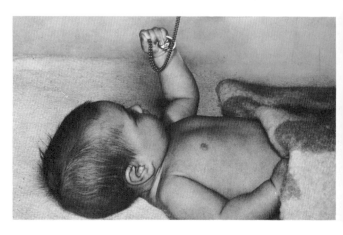

accepts and holds objects

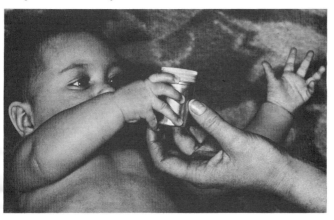

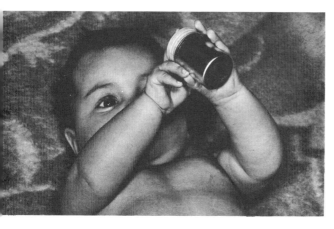

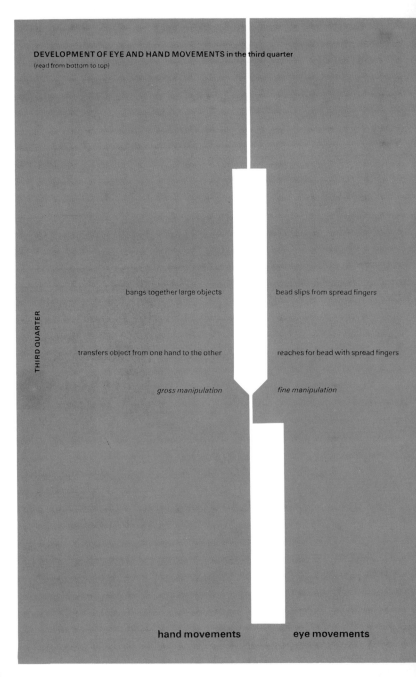

DEVELOPMENT OF EYE AND HAND MOVEMENTS in the third quarter
(read from bottom to top)

THIRD QUARTER

bangs together large objects

transfers object from one hand to the other

gross manipulation

bead slips from spread fingers

reaches for bead with spread fingers

fine manipulation

hand movements

eye movements

Third quarter

At the beginning of the third quarter the infant is able to pick up cubes and transfer them from one hand to the other, or hold one cube in each hand.

Manipulation of small objects, however, like beads or marbles, still causes difficulties. With fingers spread out like scissors, the child attempts, but fails, to pick up a marble. These attempts are repeated but with continuing lack of success; the only result is that the marble rolls about.

In the course of the third quarter, however, manual skill increases, especially as far as the manipulation of relatively large objects is concerned. Toys are banged together and thrown on the floor. Marbles still slip from between the fingers when an attempt is made to pick them up.

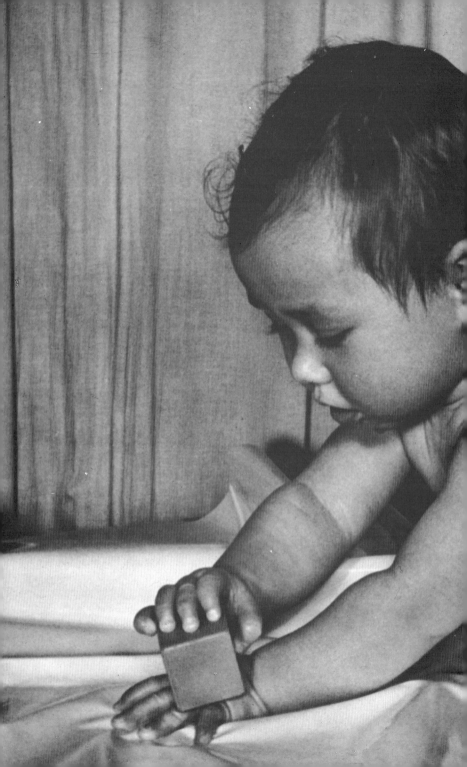

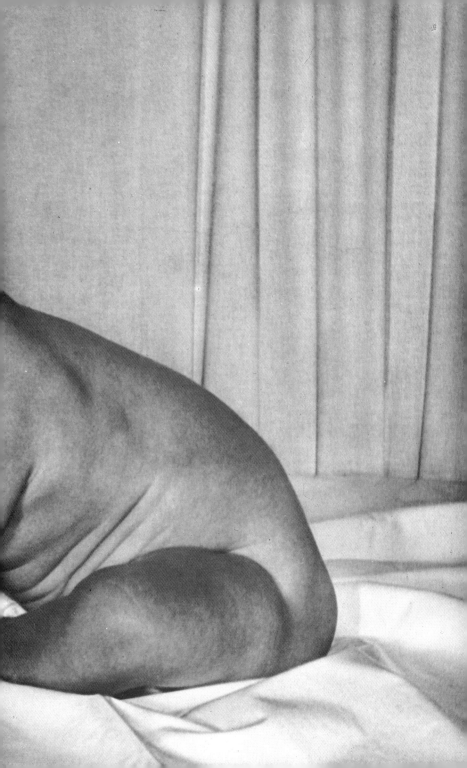

fine manipulation
rakes at marble with
"scissor-like" movements

gross manipulation
picks up cube

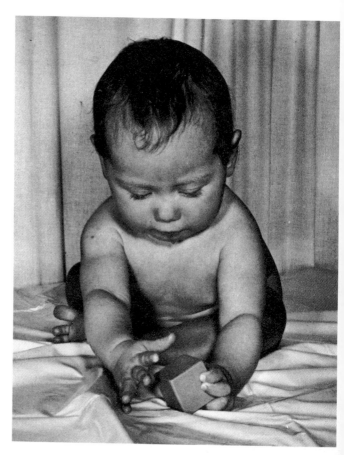

100

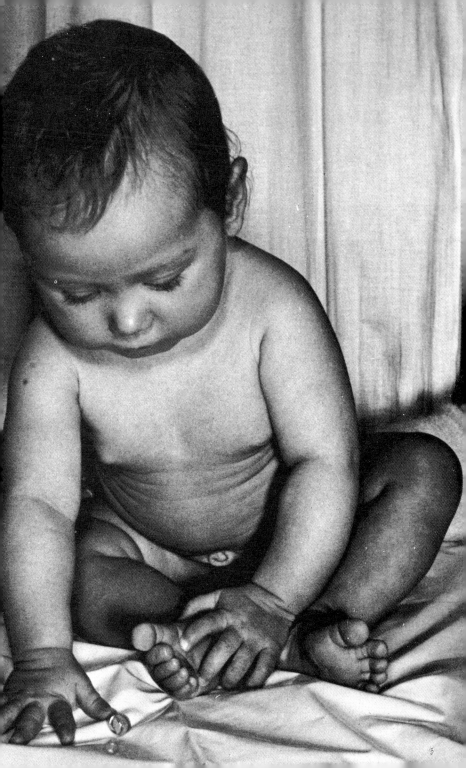

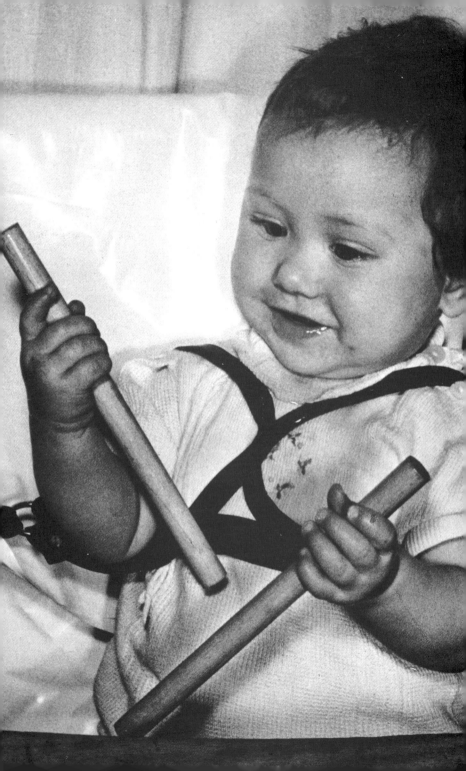

gross manipulation
handles large objects

fine manipulation
marble slips between spread fingers

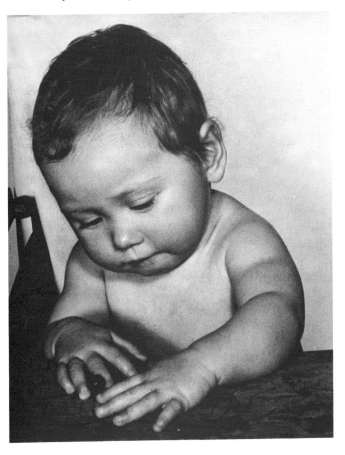

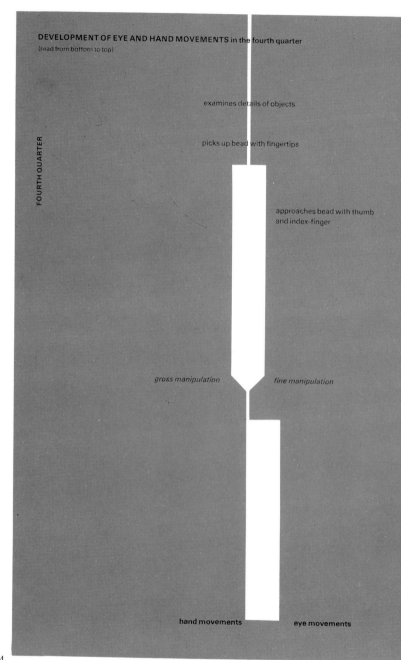

DEVELOPMENT OF EYE AND HAND MOVEMENTS in the fourth quarter
(read from bottom to top)

FOURTH QUARTER

examines details of objects

picks up bead with fingertips

approaches bead with thumb
and index-finger

gross manipulation   *fine manipulation*

hand movements   **eye movements**

Fourth quarter

At the beginning of the fourth quarter the child attempts to pick up marbles between thumb and index-finger. This is not yet completely successful; the movements are still uncertain.

In the course of the fourth quarter manual skill increases considerably. Marbles and beads are now picked up by the tips of the thumb and index-finger and can be returned to his outstretched hand.

Around the first birthday the child's play with cubes becomes more purposeful. Details of objects are examined with the finger-tips. Objects are no longer clenched in the whole hand but held by the finger-tips.

The second half year is not only characterized by the transition from sitting to crawling and walking but also by an increasing co-ordination of eye and hand movements leading to more skilled manipulation.

fine manipulation

above: marble picked up and held rather uncertainly
below: picks up marble between the tips of thumb and index-finger

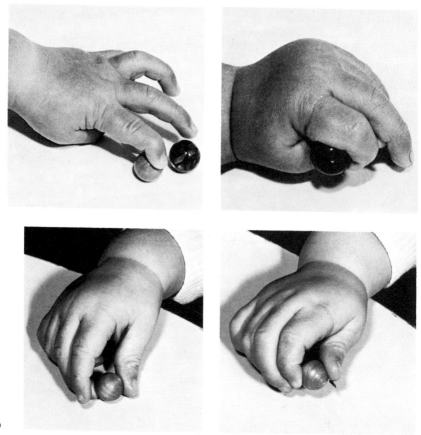

above: marble is lost between fingers
below: marble is transferred from one hand to the other

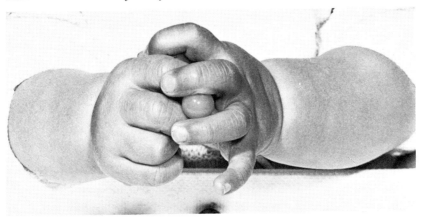

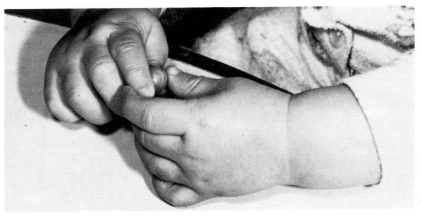

co-ordination of fine and gross manipulation

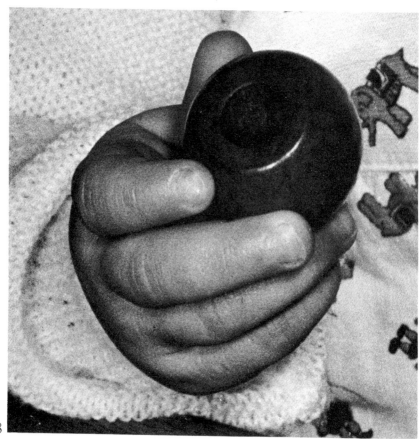

examines details of objects by touch

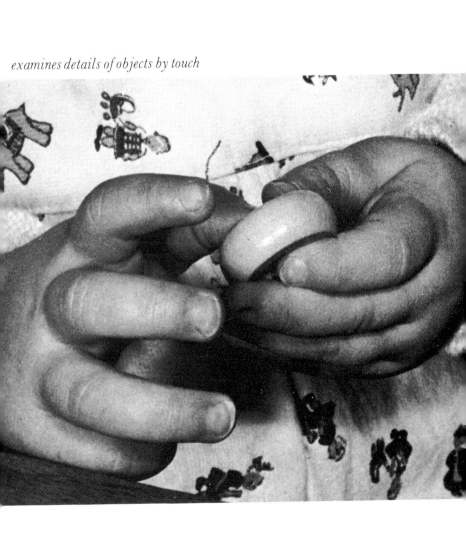

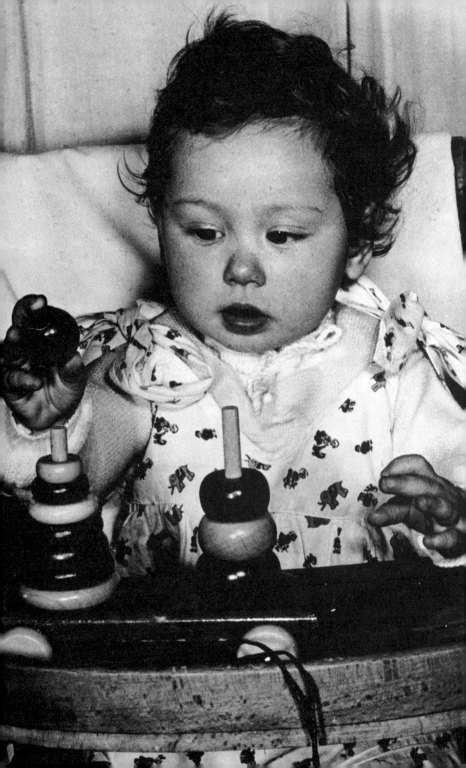

Eating and Drinking during the first year of life

GROWTH DURING THE FIRST YEAR OF LIFE bi-monthly increments

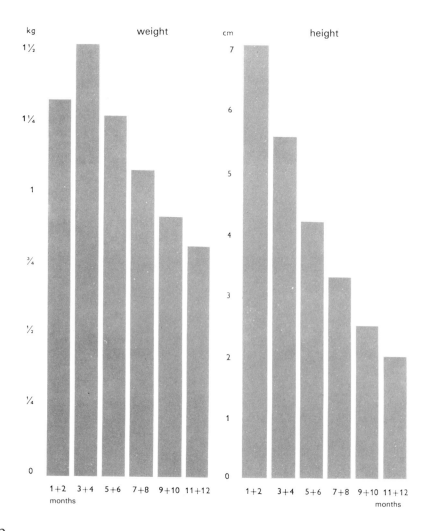

Eating and drinking during the first year of life

The photographs of motor functions tend to accentuate development more than growth.

Development is defined as the continually increasing complexity of functions and growth as the increase in the size of the body and its organs.

Growth and development are inseparably connected and only possible if sufficient food of correct composition is available. When this is the case and if the child receives the necessary attention, the average infant will tend to develop as is indicated in the growth diagrams and the photographs.

No binding conclusions as to the advance or retardation of development in any individual child can be drawn from comparison with these examples.

The child needs food and therefore has to be able to eat and drink. These functions develop according to a certain pattern.

After birth the sucking reflex makes breast or bottle feeding possible. After a few days the new-born baby is able to ingest an adequate amount of fluid and to convert mother- or cow-milk into the elements necessary for growth.

The sucking at breast or bottle is mainly reflex during the first quarter. In the transition to the second quarter the child actively participates in drinking (from a cup) and eating (from a spoon).

The transition from liquid to solid food is not very marked.

In the third quarter the child starts to hold the cup by himself and brings solid food to his mouth.

At the end of the first year the future toddler wants to help himself to food and resents help from others.

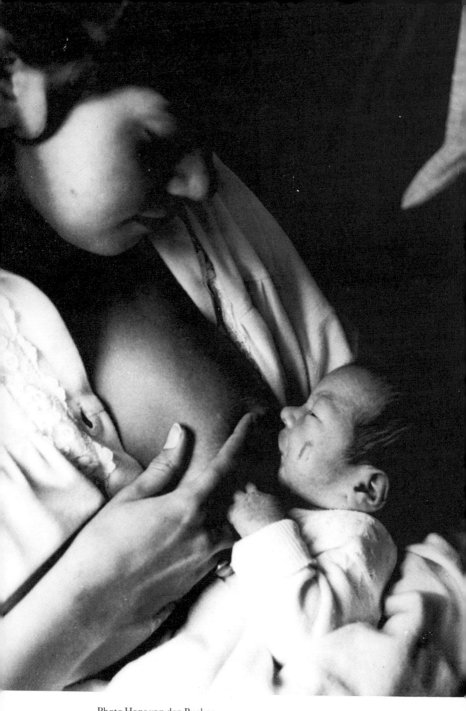

Photo Hans van den Busken

above: breast feeding
below: bottle feeding

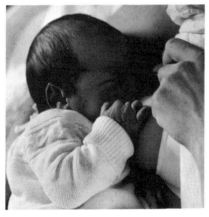

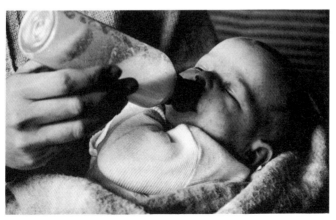

breast and supplementary feeding

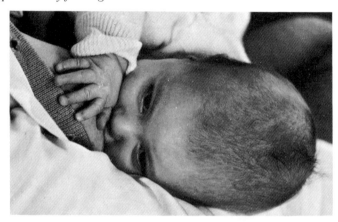

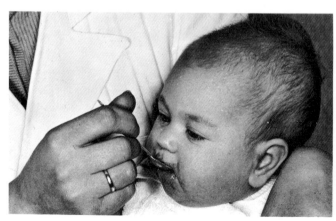

learns to drink from a cup

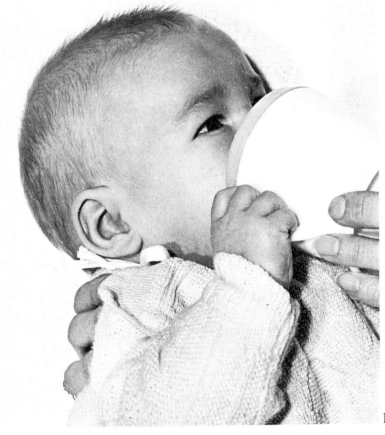

drinks from cup (assisted)

eats a biscuit unassisted

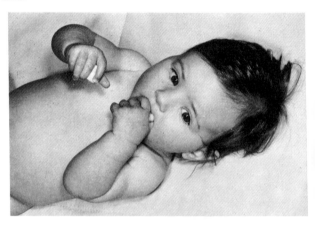

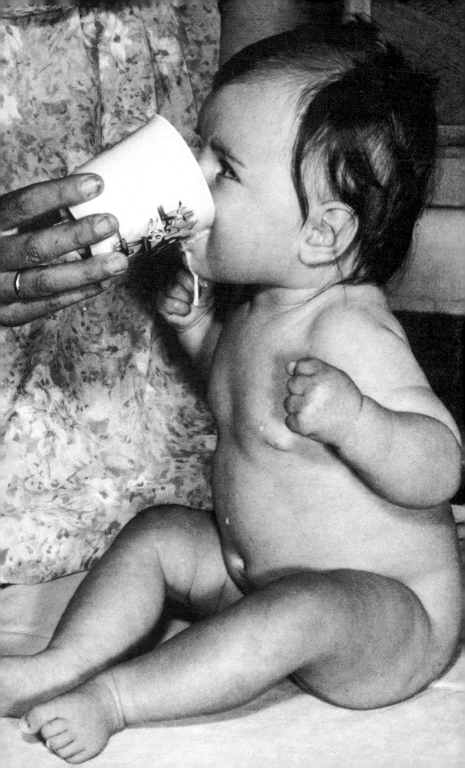

attempts to drink from a cup unaided

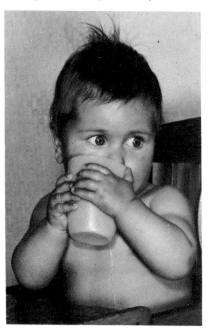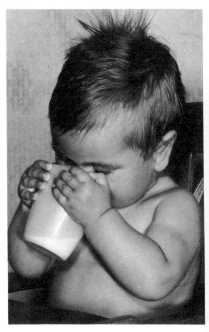

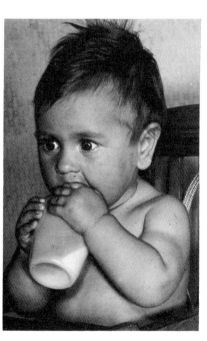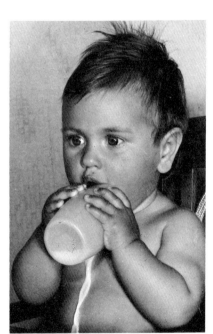

attempts unaided spoon feeding

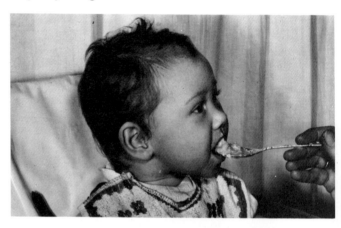

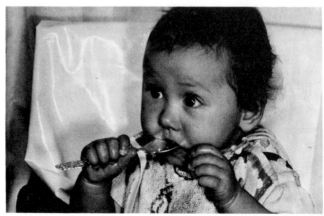

turns spoon around in mouth

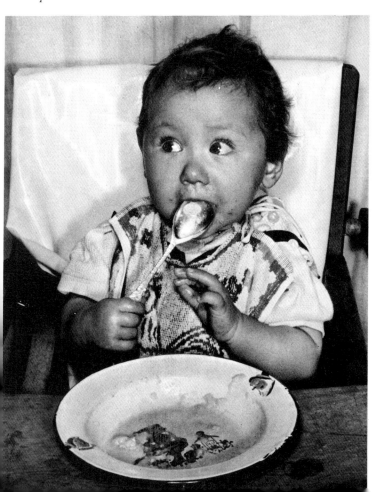

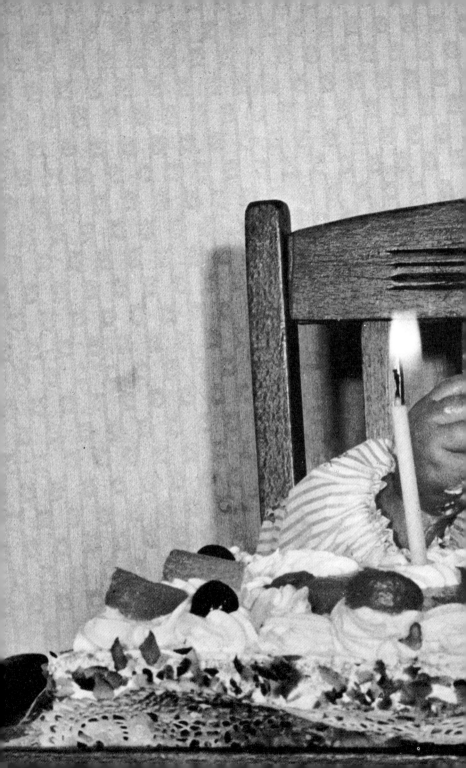

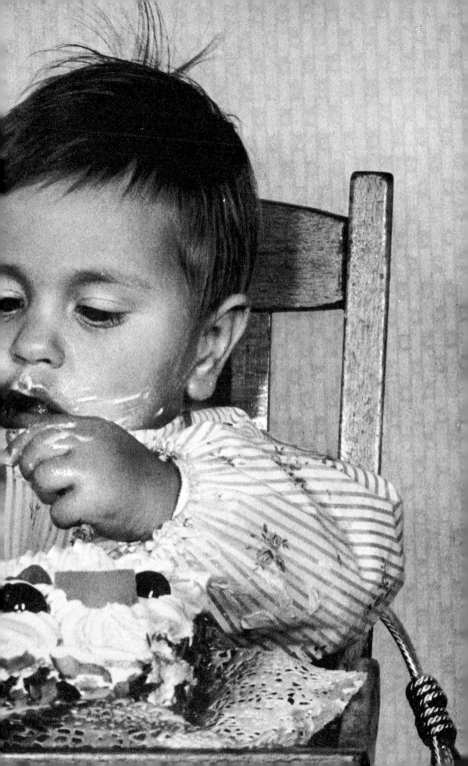

PARENTS' NOTES

name of child						
STEPPING STONES OF DEVELOPMENT	date	age in months	date	age in months	date	age in months
birth						
first visit infant welfare clinic						
first smile						
raises head in prone position						
rolls on side						
rolls from side to back						
rolls from supine to prone						
sits supported						
sits unsupported						
begins to crawl						
stands supported						
stands unsupported						
walks along play-pen						
walks supported by one hand						
walks free						

FIRST TEETH

when a tooth erupts fill in date

upper / lower — right / left (three sets)